# Gastroparesis Diet Food List

### Nourishing Your Body: A Comprehensive Guide to the Gastroparesis Nutrition Plan

McDonnell B. Young

# Table of Contents

# Introduction



In the quaint town of Elmswood, where everyone knew each other's names and business, Janet Murphy stood out—not just for her vibrant personality but also for her struggle with a condition few understood: gastroparesis. After years of battling unpredictable symptoms, her discovery of the "Gastroparesis Diet Food List" guide turned a new leaf in her life, one she was eager to share at the town's annual health fair.

The morning was bright and clear as Janet set up her booth, adorned with colorful banners reading, "Unlock the Secret to Managing Gastroparesis!" Stacks of the guidebook, her newfound treasure, were neatly arranged on the table. Curious townsfolk meandered over, drawn by the promise of relief that twinkled in Janet's eyes—a spark that had been absent for too long.

"Why this book?" asked a young woman, cradling a newborn. "I've tried so many things for my digestion issues."

Janet's smile was gentle, empathetic. "Let me tell you a story," she began, her voice tinged with a mix of nostalgia and triumph. "Just six months ago, I was where you might be now—confused and often in pain after meals, battling nausea and fatigue that wouldn't let up. Doctors said, 'gastroparesis,' but that diagnosis only led to more questions than answers."

She picked up a copy of the guide. "This isn't just a book; it's a roadmap. Each chapter is crafted to not only tell you what you can and cannot eat but also why. For those of us with gastroparesis, understanding the 'why' can make all the difference."

Janet flipped the book open to a marked page. "See here," she pointed at a colorful chart. "It lists foods that are generally safe—like well-cooked carrots and chicken broth. And over here," she flipped a few pages, "are the ones to avoid, like raw apples and carbonated drinks, which can aggravate our symptoms."

The woman listened, nodding as she bounced her baby lightly. "But how has it really changed things for you?" she asked, a hint of skepticism in her voice.

"That's the best part," Janet exclaimed. Her energy was infectious. "By following the dietary guidelines here, my flare-ups have reduced significantly. I'm not just eating blindly; I'm choosing foods that my stomach can handle. It means fewer days spent in bed, more days out here, enjoying life."

She gestured around the fair, her gaze settling on the laughing children and chatting neighbors. "This guide taught me how to adjust not just what I eat, but how and when. Small, frequent meals, nothing too fibrous or fatty. It even includes tips for managing symptoms when they do arise, like natural remedies and hydration techniques."

The young mother was visibly moved, her initial skepticism giving way to a hopeful curiosity. "It sounds like it's given you back control," she murmured.

"Exactly," Janet confirmed, her voice firm. "Control, and with it, a slice of my life I thought I'd lost. I can't promise miracles, but for anyone struggling with gastroparesis, this guide is a solid foundation. It's practical, easy to understand, and most importantly, it's effective."

As the day wore on, Janet shared her story with many more visitors, each conversation adding to a growing buzz around her booth. Copies of the "Gastroparesis Diet Food List" guide began to disappear into eager hands, each sale a beacon of hope.

By the fair's end, as Janet packed up her now sparse table, she felt a warmth that went beyond the afternoon sun. In sharing her journey and the guide that changed it, she had not only spread awareness but had also kindled a flame of community support and understanding—something every heart in Elmswood could cherish.

# Understanding the Importance of Diet Management

Gastroparesis is a condition characterized by delayed gastric emptying, where the stomach takes too long to empty its contents. This disorder affects the normal spontaneous movement of the muscles in your stomach, often leading to a range of symptoms such as nausea, vomiting, abdominal bloating, and feeling full quickly after starting a meal. The management of gastroparesis primarily focuses on dietary adjustments to ease these symptoms and improve gastric motility. By understanding the types of foods that are more easily digested, individuals with gastroparesis can tailor their diets to minimize discomfort and enhance their quality of life.

Soft, well-cooked fruits and vegetables are typically recommended for those with gastroparesis. This is because raw fruits and vegetables contain fibrous materials that can be hard to digest and may form bezoars in the stomach, which are trapped masses that can exacerbate symptoms. Cooking helps break down some of the fibers, making these foods gentler on the stomach. However, even cooked, some vegetables like broccoli, corn, and cabbage are high in insoluble fiber and should be avoided.

Lean proteins such as chicken, turkey, and fish are often more easily tolerated by individuals with gastroparesis. These foods provide necessary nutrients without the high fat content that can slow gastric emptying. Fatty meats and fried foods can exacerbate gastroparesis symptoms by delaying stomach emptying and should be consumed minimally. Similarly, while protein is crucial, care must be taken to prepare these items in a way that makes them as easy to digest as possible, such as grilling or baking rather than frying.

Carbohydrates that are low in fiber and fat are also an essential component of the gastroparesis diet. Options like white bread, white rice, and specially formulated low-fiber cereals can be beneficial. These foods provide energy without the risk of fiber-induced delays in stomach emptying. However, patients should be wary of sugars and refined carbs that can lead to spikes in blood sugar, which is particularly important for those who also have diabetes, a common comorbidity with gastroparesis.

Hydration is crucial for managing gastroparesis, but the type of fluids consumed can also impact symptoms. Water is always a good option, yet sometimes, beverages with electrolytes might be necessary to prevent dehydration, especially if vomiting is a frequent symptom. Carbonated beverages and alcoholic drinks should be avoided as they can trigger further stomach discomfort and contribute to dehydration.

The consistency of food can play a significant role in how well it is tolerated. Smoothies, soups, and purees can be particularly beneficial for a gastroparesis diet as they are easier to digest. These can also be nutritious ways to incorporate fruits, vegetables, and proteins into the diet without the bulk of fiber. Meals should be small and frequent rather than large and overwhelming to the digestive system, which helps in managing the volume of food that the stomach has to handle at any given time.

It is also important for individuals with gastroparesis to monitor their diet's impact on their symptoms and adjust accordingly. What works for one person may not work for another, so tailoring the diet to individual needs and reactions is crucial. Consulting with a dietitian who specializes in gastroparesis can help in developing a meal plan that not only manages symptoms but also ensures nutritional balance. This partnership can be essential in managing the condition effectively, as the dietitian can provide ongoing support and adjustments based on the progression of symptoms or response to the initial diet plan.

# Chapter 1: Basics of Gastroparesis

## What is Gastroparesis?

Gastroparesis is a chronic medical condition where the stomach's ability to empty itself is impaired, not due to any obstruction but because of a problem with the nerves and muscles that control the stomach's motility. In a healthy digestive system, strong muscular contractions push food through the digestive tract. But in gastroparesis, these contractions are weak or irregular, which can lead to a variety of symptoms including nausea, vomiting, acid reflux, and feeling full quickly after starting a meal. This condition can significantly impact quality of life by causing malnutrition, unintentional weight loss, and poor blood sugar control in people with diabetes.

The exact cause of gastroparesis is not always clear, but it is often associated with other health conditions. Diabetes is a common link because high blood sugar levels can damage the vagus nerve, which controls the stomach muscles. Other possible causes include surgeries that involve the digestive system, certain medications that affect muscle action in the intestine, and conditions such as Parkinson's disease and multiple sclerosis. In many cases, however, gastroparesis appears without a known cause, termed idiopathic gastroparesis.

Symptoms of gastroparesis can vary in severity and may come and go. The most common symptoms include nausea and vomiting, especially of undigested food; a bloated feeling after eating; lack of appetite; and stomach pain. These symptoms not only make it difficult to eat a normal meal, which can affect a person's nutritional and metabolic status, but can also impact emotional and psychological well-being due to the chronic nature of the illness and the dietary restrictions it imposes.

Managing gastroparesis often requires a combination of dietary changes, medications, and sometimes surgical interventions. Dietary management is critical and focuses on modifying the diet to ensure that food moves through the stomach more easily. Patients are advised to eat small, frequent meals that are low in fats and fibers, both of which can slow stomach emptying. Liquids and soft foods, such as soups and purees, are often recommended because they require less gastric processing and are less likely to cause discomfort.

Specific foods are recommended for those with gastroparesis. Soft, well-cooked fruits and vegetables are easier for the stomach to digest compared to raw ones. Lean meats, such as skinless poultry or fish, provide necessary proteins without adding a lot of fat that could delay stomach emptying. Low-fiber starches like white rice, white bread, and potatoes without the skin are also easier to digest. These foods form the basis of the gastroparesis diet and can help manage symptoms by facilitating smoother digestion and reducing the risk of food being regurgitated.

Fluid intake is also a crucial aspect of managing gastroparesis, as it helps ensure that nutrients move through the system and can help prevent dehydration due to vomiting. Patients are encouraged to drink non-carbonated, low-fat, and low-fiber fluids between meals. Care must be taken with certain beverages like alcohol or caffeinated drinks, which can exacerbate symptoms. Some patients might also benefit from nutritional supplements, especially if their caloric intake is compromised.

Overall, while gastroparesis can be a challenging and often frustrating condition, careful dietary management can greatly enhance a patient's quality of life. Working closely with a healthcare provider or a dietitian to tailor a diet plan that fits one's specific nutritional needs and symptom profile is essential. As each individual's response to different foods can vary widely, personal experience with certain foods can also guide dietary choices to better manage the condition.

# Symptoms and Diagnosis

Gastroparesis is often recognized by its distinctive symptoms that arise from the inefficient movement of the stomach muscles. Among the most common symptoms is nausea, which can vary from mild to severe and may or may not lead to vomiting. Vomiting, when it occurs, typically happens after eating as the delayed gastric emptying prevents normal digestion. This symptom can lead to dehydration and malnutrition if not managed properly. Patients frequently experience abdominal bloating and pain, which result from the buildup of undigested food in the stomach. These symptoms can be exacerbated by certain foods, highlighting the need for a carefully managed diet.

Feeling full quickly while eating is another hallmark symptom of gastroparesis. This sensation, known as early satiety, can make it difficult to consume enough calories and nutrients, as patients feel full after eating only small amounts of food. This can complicate efforts to maintain a balanced diet and may require dietary adjustments to ensure sufficient nutrient intake. Weight loss often occurs as a result of reduced calorie intake and is a significant concern that needs to be addressed in dietary planning.

Sufferers of gastroparesis may also experience fluctuations in blood sugar levels. For those with diabetes, gastroparesis can complicate blood sugar management because delayed gastric emptying affects the timing of glucose absorption and insulin administration. This interplay between diabetes and gastroparesis necessitates careful monitoring and adjustment of both insulin therapy and meal planning to prevent either hypo- or hyperglycemia.

The diagnosis of gastroparesis typically begins with a review of the patient's medical history and a physical examination, focusing on symptoms and dietary habits. Physicians may inquire about the types and severity of symptoms, their relation to meals, and any patterns noticed by the patient. This initial assessment helps to rule out other conditions that could mimic gastroparesis, such as peptic ulcers or stomach cancers.

To confirm a diagnosis of gastroparesis, a gastric emptying study is often performed. This test measures the speed at which food leaves the stomach and enters the small intestine. Patients eat a meal that includes a small amount of radioactive material, and a scanner tracks the rate of digestion. Results that show food remains in the stomach longer than normal can confirm the presence of gastroparesis.

Additional diagnostic tests might include an upper gastrointestinal endoscopy to rule out physical blockages that could impede stomach emptying. This procedure involves using a flexible tube with a camera to view the upper digestive system. Doctors may also perform tests to evaluate stomach and small bowel motility and function, providing comprehensive insights into the digestive process and identifying any abnormalities that might contribute to symptoms.

Managing the symptoms of gastroparesis often involves a specialized diet designed to minimize the workload on the stomach. This diet typically includes foods that are easy to digest and low in fat and fiber. Small, frequent meals and plenty of fluids are recommended to aid digestion and prevent dehydration. Patients are advised to avoid raw fruits and vegetables, high-fiber foods, and fatty meals, as these can exacerbate symptoms. Nutritional supplements may also be recommended to ensure adequate nutrient intake, especially if weight loss has been significant. Regular follow-ups with healthcare providers are essential to monitor the condition and adjust dietary guidelines as needed to manage symptoms effectively.

# How Diet Influences Gastroparesis

Gastroparesis, a chronic condition where the stomach is unable to empty properly, has profound implications on digestion and overall health. The symptoms—ranging from nausea and vomiting to bloating and early satiety—can significantly impair quality of life. One of the primary management strategies for gastroparesis involves dietary modifications, as certain foods can exacerbate symptoms while others may alleviate them. The relationship between diet and gastroparesis management is both intricate and individualized, requiring a well-considered approach to food choices and meal timing.

For people with gastroparesis, foods that are high in fats and fibers pose particular challenges. Fatty foods slow down gastric emptying, which can worsen symptoms like fullness and nausea. Similarly, high-fiber foods can be difficult to digest and may lead to the formation of bezoars—hardened masses of undigested material that can block the gastrointestinal tract. Therefore, the gastroparesis diet typically recommends low-fat and low-fiber foods to help minimize these risks and promote easier gastric processing.

The types of carbohydrates chosen are crucial in managing gastroparesis. Simple carbohydrates, which are found in foods like white bread, white rice, and potatoes, can be easier for the stomach to digest. These foods are less likely to cause distress than complex carbohydrates found in whole grains and raw fruits and vegetables. However, it is important to balance carbohydrate intake with other nutrients to avoid rapid spikes in blood sugar, especially in patients who are also diabetic—a common condition co-occurring with gastroparesis.

Lean protein sources such as chicken, turkey, and fish are generally recommended because they provide essential nutrients without the high fat content that can aggravate gastroparesis. These proteins should be prepared in ways that minimize fat content, such as baking or poaching, rather than frying. Incorporating these proteins into a gastroparesis diet helps maintain muscle mass and strength, which is vital as the condition can often lead to malnutrition due to poor digestion and reduced appetite.

The physical form of food can also impact how well it is tolerated. Pureed and liquid foods, such as smoothies and soups, are often easier to digest. These forms reduce the work that the compromised stomach has to do to break down food, potentially reducing symptoms like nausea and vomiting. For many with severe gastroparesis, these may constitute a significant portion of the diet, especially during flare-ups when symptoms are more pronounced.

Meal frequency and size are important considerations in the management of gastroparesis. Smaller, more frequent meals can help by putting less strain on the stomach at any one time. Large meals can overwhelm the stomach, exacerbating symptoms and discomfort. Timing meals to allow several hours of digestion before lying down can also help reduce symptoms like heartburn and regurgitation, as gravity assists in the movement of food through the digestive system.

Ultimately, managing gastroparesis with diet is highly personalized. Patients often benefit from working with a dietitian who specializes in digestive disorders to tailor their food choices to their specific needs. This professional can help devise a plan that not only fits the patient's nutritional requirements and lifestyle but also adapates to their changing symptoms. Regular follow-ups and adjustments to the diet plan are crucial, as gastroparesis can vary over time, and what works initially may need to be modified as the condition progresses or improves.

# Chapter 2: General Dietary Guidelines for Gastroparesis

## Principles of a Gastroparesis Diet

Gastroparesis requires a tailored approach to diet due to the stomach's impaired ability to empty effectively. People dealing with this condition need to choose foods that minimize symptoms and support easier digestion. The primary focus is on consuming meals that can pass through the stomach more swiftly and without causing distress. This involves selecting foods that are low in fiber and fat, as these two components are known to slow gastric emptying. Processed grains like white bread, white rice, and low-fiber cereals are often recommended because they are less likely to form indigestible masses that can exacerbate symptoms.

Protein is essential in any diet but requires careful consideration in a gastroparesis diet. Lean proteins such as poultry, fish, and eggs are preferable because they provide the necessary nutrients without the high fat content that can aggravate the condition. Cooking methods should be aimed at making these proteins as easy to digest as possible; grilled or baked options are typically better than fried ones. Patients must be cautious with meats that are tough or fatty, as these can be particularly challenging for the stomach to process.

The texture of food is crucial in managing gastroparesis. Pureed or blended foods are often easier to digest. These might include smoothies made from low-fiber fruits and vegetables or soups that are smooth and free from chunks of food. This approach not only ensures that nutrients are more readily available but also helps in keeping the stomach from becoming overly full, which can trigger symptoms like nausea and vomiting. Small, frequent meals are recommended over larger, heavier meals to keep the digestive process manageable.

Hydration is another key component of the gastroparesis diet, but not all fluids are equally beneficial. Water is excellent for maintaining hydration, but some patients may need to supplement with electrolyte solutions, especially if symptoms like vomiting or diarrhea occur frequently. It is important to avoid alcoholic beverages and drinks that are carbonated or very high in sugar, as these can disrupt digestion and cause additional bloating and discomfort.

Certain fruits and vegetables can be included in a gastroparesis diet, but care must be taken with selection and preparation. Cooked fruits and vegetables are often more digestible than raw ones. However, even among cooked options, choices like applesauce or canned peaches are preferable to fibrous options like oranges or broccoli. These selections are based on the fiber content and the physical properties of the food after cooking, which can impact how easily they are digested.

Avoiding fats is particularly important in a gastroparesis diet because fat slows down the digestive process. This doesn't just apply to fatty cuts of meat but also to cooking oils, butter, and high-fat dairy products. Patients should aim to prepare foods without added fats and choose low-fat or fat-free options where available to help facilitate easier digestion.

Finally, individual response to different foods can vary significantly among those with gastroparesis, making personalized diet planning essential. Regular consultation with a dietitian or a healthcare provider specialized in digestive disorders is important to tailor the diet to individual needs. This professional guidance ensures that not only are the symptoms managed effectively, but nutritional needs are also met to support overall health and well-being.

# The Role of Dietitians and Nutritionists

Dietitians and nutritionists play a pivotal role in managing gastroparesis, a condition that affects the normal movement of the stomach muscles and results in delayed emptying of stomach contents. These professionals help in crafting personalized diet plans based on the severity of symptoms and individual nutritional needs, guiding patients through the complex process of selecting appropriate foods that can be digested more easily. Their expertise is critical in ensuring that patients receive balanced nutrition while managing the specific challenges posed by gastroparesis, such as malnutrition, dehydration, and avoidance of certain fibers that exacerbate symptoms.

In managing gastroparesis, dietitians and nutritionists often recommend a diet low in fats and fibers, which are harder for the stomach to process. High-fat foods slow down gastric emptying, and high-fiber foods can lead to the formation of bezoars—hardened masses of food that block the stomach outlet. Thus, they advise on the consumption of cooked, rather than raw, fruits and vegetables, as cooking breaks down the fibers making them easier to digest. Similarly, they suggest skinless and seedless varieties to minimize fiber intake.

Protein intake is crucial, but the type of protein selected is key. Dietitians typically recommend easily digestible proteins, such as low-fat poultry, fish, eggs, and tofu. These provide essential nutrients without contributing to the slow-down of gastric processing. Preparing these proteins through boiling, poaching, or grilling rather than frying helps avoid unnecessary fat which can aggravate gastroparesis symptoms.

Carbohydrates are a significant part of the diet but should be chosen carefully. Simple carbohydrates such as white bread, rice, and low-fiber cereals are usually recommended because they are less likely to cause distress. These foods provide the needed calories and are generally easier to digest, helping to maintain energy levels without stressing the stomach. However, nutritionists also caution against the excessive intake of sugary foods to prevent spikes in blood sugar levels, particularly in gastroparesis patients who also have diabetes.

Regarding fluids, maintaining adequate hydration is essential, especially for those who frequently experience vomiting as a symptom of gastroparesis. Dietitians often emphasize the importance of drinking small amounts of fluids throughout the day. Non-carbonated, non-caffeinated, and low-fat beverages are preferred to minimize irritation to the stomach. In some cases, they may recommend meal replacement drinks or supplements to ensure nutritional needs are met without overwhelming the stomach.

Meal timing and frequency are also adjusted according to the individual's tolerance. Small, frequent meals are usually easier to manage than large meals, as they require less gastric effort and minimize symptoms. Dietitians work closely with patients to develop eating schedules that align with their energy needs and daily routines, adjusting as necessary based on how well food is tolerated and the progression of symptoms.

The ongoing relationship between a patient with gastroparesis and their dietitian or nutritionist is dynamic and requires regular adjustments and monitoring. This collaboration is key to finding the most effective and sustainable dietary strategy to manage symptoms and maintain health. As gastroparesis can significantly impact quality of life, the support and guidance from these nutritional experts are invaluable in helping patients adapt to lifestyle changes and achieve the best possible outcomes with their diet.

# Meal Planning and Frequency

Meal planning and frequency are pivotal aspects of managing gastroparesis, a condition characterized by the stomach's inability to empty efficiently. Those dealing with this condition must carefully consider not only what they eat but also how often and in what quantities. Smaller, more frequent meals can prevent the stomach from becoming too full, which can exacerbate symptoms like nausea and vomiting. Typically, six small meals a day are recommended over three larger ones. This frequent eating schedule helps maintain a steady movement through the stomach, easing the workload on the digestive system.

The composition of these meals plays a critical role in their effectiveness. Meals high in fats and fibers are harder to digest, which can be particularly challenging for individuals with gastroparesis. Instead, meals should be based on foods that are easier to digest, such as low-fiber fruits and vegetables and lean proteins. Preparing these foods in a way that further aids digestion, such as blending or cooking them thoroughly, can also make a significant difference. For instance, turning fruits into smoothies or cooking vegetables until they are soft helps minimize the effort required by the stomach to process them.

Starches and grains are an essential component of any diet but should be chosen wisely in the context of gastroparesis. Refined grains such as white rice, white bread, and pasta are usually better tolerated than their whole-grain counterparts because they are lower in fiber. These should be cooked until very soft to ensure they are as easy as possible for the stomach to handle. The simplicity of these foods helps in maintaining an energy supply without causing significant delays in gastric emptying.

Proteins are crucial but should be consumed in forms that are easy to digest to prevent exacerbating gastroparesis symptoms. Lean meats such as poultry, fish, or eggs are excellent choices. These proteins should be prepared grilled, baked, or poached rather than fried or in rich, fatty sauces. Dairy products can also be part of the diet, but low-fat or fat-free options are preferable, as fat can slow stomach emptying. In cases where solid proteins are difficult to tolerate, protein shakes or smoothies may be used as substitutes.

Liquids are another essential element of meal planning for gastroparesis. Drinking enough fluids is crucial to avoid dehydration, especially for those who frequently experience vomiting as a symptom of their condition. However, fluids should be consumed separately from meals to prevent the stomach from filling too quickly. Drinking 30 minutes before or after eating solids is generally recommended. This strategy helps keep hydration levels up without increasing the volume of the stomach's contents during meals.

Adjusting meal consistency can also aid digestion. For those with severe gastroparesis, traditional solid meals may not be viable.

Instead, meals based on pureed or liquid foods can be beneficial. These might include soups, purees, and smoothies that provide necessary nutrition without requiring significant gastric processing. These should be carefully balanced to ensure that all essential nutrients are included, despite the altered form of the meals.

Lastly, personal monitoring and adjustment of the diet are key. Because gastroparesis affects individuals differently, a diet that works well for one person may not be effective for another. Keeping a food diary to track what foods and meal schedules work best can be incredibly useful. Regular consultations with a healthcare provider or dietitian specialized in digestive disorders can ensure the diet remains appropriate and beneficial as symptoms change or improve. Tailoring the diet to personal tolerances and reactions is crucial for managing gastroparesis effectively and maintaining overall health and well-being.

# Chapter 3: Foods to Eat

## Nutritional Considerations

Below is a table outlining 15 nutritional considerations for individuals managing gastroparesis, focusing on food groups that are generally recommended due to their easier digestibility. The table includes ingredients, instructions for preparation, nutritional information, recommended serving sizes, and estimated cooking times.

| Ingredient | Preparation Instructions | Nutritional Information per Serving | Serving Size | Cooking Time |
| --- | --- | --- | --- | --- |
| Cooked Carrot | Steam or boil until very soft. Puree for easier digestion. | 55 calories, 0.1g fat, 1.2g protein | ½ cup | 10-15 minutes |

| Baked Chicken Breast | Bake with light seasoning. Avoid skin and fats. | 165 calories, 3.6g fat, 31g protein | 3 ounces | 20-25 minutes |
|---|---|---|---|---|
| White Rice | Cook with water until soft and fluffy. | 205 calories, 0.4g fat, 4.3g protein | 1 cup cooked | 18-20 minutes |
| Banana Smoothie | Blend ripe bananas with a splash of lactose-fre e milk. | 150 calories, 0.2g fat, 1.9g protein | 1 medium glass | 5 minutes |
| Apple Sauce | Cook peeled apples until soft, blend to smooth | 100 calories, 0.2g fat, 0.5g protein | ½ cup | 15-20 minutes |

| | consistency. | | | |
| --- | --- | --- | --- | --- |
| Poached Fish | Poach in water or broth until fish flakes easily. | 85 calories, 1g fat, 18g protein | 3 ounces | 10-15 minutes |
| Scrambled Eggs | Lightly scramble eggs with a bit of olive oil or water. | 91 calories, 7g fat, 6g protein | 1 large egg | 3-5 minutes |
| Oatmeal (Instant) | Cook instant oatmeal with water until soft. | 158 calories, 3.2g fat, 4g protein | 1 packet | 1-2 minutes |
| Avocado Puree | Puree ripe avocado with a | 240 calories, | ½ medium avocado | 5 minutes |

| | | | | |
|---|---|---|---|---|
| | pinch of salt. | 22g fat, 3g protein | | |
| Mashed Potatoes | Boil potatoes until soft, mash with lactose-fre e milk. | 160 calories, 0.2g fat, 4g protein | ½ cup | 20-25 minutes |
| Tofu | Steam or lightly sauté until warm. Serve soft. | 70 calories, 4g fat, 8g protein | 3 ounces | 5-10 minutes |
| Custard | Cook low-fat milk with eggs and sugar until thick. | 120 calories, 3g fat, 5g protein | ½ cup | 10 minutes |
| Rice Porridge | Cook rice in excess water | 150 calories, 0.3g fat, | 1 cup | 25-30 minutes |

| | until very soft and porridge-like. | 3.1g protein | | |
|---|---|---|---|---|
| Cottage Cheese | Serve plain or blended for smoother consistency. | 206 calories, 9.7g fat, 23g protein | ½ cup | No cooking |
| Gelatin (Flavored) | Dissolve gelatin in hot water, refrigerate until set. | 70 calories, 0g fat, 1g protein | ½ cup | 1-2 hours (chill) |

Each of these foods has been selected based on its ease of digestion and lower fiber content, making them suitable options for those with gastroparesis. Preparation methods are aimed at making the foods as soft and easy to digest as possible. Nutritional values are approximate and can vary based on specific brands or exact ingredients used.

# Safe Foods List

Here's a detailed table listing safe foods for individuals managing gastroparesis, including specific ingredients, instructions for preparation, nutritional information, serving size, and cooking time:

| Food Item | Ingredient | Preparation Instruction | Nutritional Information per Serving | Serving Size | Cooking Time |
|---|---|---|---|---|---|
| Cooked Carrot Soup | Carrots | Peel and boil carrots until soft, blend to puree | 45 calories, 1g protein, 0g fat | 1 cup | 30 minutes |
| Mashed Potatoes | Potatoes | Boil peeled potatoe | 150 calories, 2g | 1/2 cup | 20 minutes |

| | | s, mash with a bit of milk | protein, 0.5g fat | | |
|---|---|---|---|---|---|
| Poached Chicken Breast | Chicken breast | Poach chicken in water or broth until cooked | 120 calories, 26g protein, 1g fat | 3 ounces | 15 minutes |
| Baked Tilapia | Tilapia | Bake tilapia with a sprinkle of herbs | 110 calories, 23g protein, 2g fat | 3 ounces | 12-15 minutes |
| Applesauce | Apples | Cook peeled apples until soft, blend to puree | 90 calories, 0g protein, 0g fat | 1/2 cup | 25 minutes |

| White Bread Toast | White bread | Toast bread lightly | 70 calories, 2g protein, 1g fat | 1 slice | 2 minutes |
|---|---|---|---|---|---|
| Rice Porridge | White rice | Cook rice in extra water until very soft | 150 calories, 3g protein, 0.4g fat | 1 cup | 20 minutes |
| Banana Smoothie | Banana | Blend ripe banana with a bit of milk or water | 120 calories, 1.5g protein, 0.3g fat | 1 cup | 5 minutes |
| Scrambled Eggs | Eggs | Scramble eggs with a dash of milk | 90 calories, 6g protein, 5g fat | 1 egg | 5 minutes |

| Plain Yogurt | Low-fat yogurt | Serve chilled | 100 calories, 9g protein, 2.5g fat | 1/2 cup | 0 minutes |
| Steamed Hake | Hake fillet | Steam fish until cooked through | 90 calories, 20g protein, 1g fat | 3 ounces | 10 minutes |
| Pureed Peas | Green peas | Cook peas until soft, blend to puree | 55 calories, 3g protein, 0g fat | 1/2 cup | 10 minutes |
| Cottage Cheese | Low-fat cottage cheese | Serve chilled | 80 calories, 14g protein, 1g fat | 1/2 cup | 0 minutes |

| Instant Oatmeal | Instant oats | Cook oats in microwave with water until soft | 130 calories, 3g protein, 2g fat | 1/2 cup | 3 minutes |
| Avocado Puree | Avocado | Blend ripe avocado until smooth | 120 calories, 2g protein, 10g fat | 1/2 avocado | 5 minutes |

These foods are chosen for their ease of digestion and low fiber content, which are crucial in managing gastroparesis effectively. The preparation methods and serving sizes are designed to minimize stomach distress while providing necessary nutrients. Cooking times are kept short to simplify meal preparation.

# Snack Ideas for Gastroparesis

Below is a detailed table presenting 15 snack ideas suitable for individuals with gastroparesis, focusing on easy digestion and minimizing symptoms. Each entry includes ingredients, simple preparation instructions, nutritional information, serving size, and estimated cooking or preparation time.

| Snack Idea | Ingredients | Instructions | Nutritional Information (approx.) | Serving Size | Cooking/Prep Time |
| --- | --- | --- | --- | --- | --- |
| 1. Avocado Smoothie | 1 ripe avocado, 1 cup almond milk, honey | Blend ingredients until smooth. | 250 calories, 15g fat | 1 cup | 5 minutes |
| 2. Banana Yogurt Pops | 1 banana, ½ cup Greek | Blend, pour into molds, freeze. | 150 calories, 1g fat | 1 pop | 4 hours (freeze) |

| | | | | | |
|---|---|---|---|---|---|
| | yogurt, honey | | | | |
| 3. Mashed Potato Cups | 2 potatoes, 1 tbsp butter, salt | Boil potatoes, mash with butter. | 200 calories, 9g fat | ½ cup | 20 minutes |
| 4. Rice Pudding | ½ cup cooked white rice, 1 cup milk, sugar | Mix ingredients, simmer until thick. | 180 calories, 2g fat | ½ cup | 15 minutes |
| 5. Applesauce | 3 apples, cinnamon, water | Cook apples with water, blend. | 100 calories, 0g fat | ½ cup | 20 minutes |
| 6. Cottage Cheese | ½ cup cottage cheese, | Mix cottage cheese | 200 calories, 2.5g fat | ½ cup | 2 minutes |

| with Honey | 1 tbsp honey | with honey. | | | |
| 7. Egg Custard | 1 egg, 1 cup milk, sugar | Beat, bake in water bath until set. | 170 calories, 10g fat | 1 serving | 45 minutes |
| 8. Peach Sorbet | 2 peaches, sugar, lemon juice | Blend ingredients, freeze. | 120 calories, 0g fat | ½ cup | 2 hours (freeze) |
| 9. Steamed Carrot Puree | 4 carrots, butter, salt | Steam carrots, puree with butter. | 90 calories, 5g fat | ½ cup | 25 minutes |
| 10. Oatmeal with Maple Syrup | ½ cup rolled oats, 1 cup water, | Cook oats, stir in syrup. | 180 calories, 2g fat | 1 cup | 10 minutes |

| | maple syrup | | | | |
| --- | --- | --- | --- | --- | --- |
| 11. Gelatin with Fruit | 1 packet gelatin, assorted fruit | Dissolve gelatin, add fruit, chill. | 70 calories, 0g fat | 1 cup | 2 hours (chill) |
| 12. Cream of Wheat | ¼ cup Cream of Wheat, 1 cup milk | Cook cereal in milk until smooth. | 150 calories, 1g fat | 1 cup | 10 minutes |
| 13. Soft Scrambled Eggs | 2 eggs, 1 tbsp milk | Gently scramble eggs with milk. | 140 calories, 10g fat | 1 serving | 5 minutes |
| 14. Baked Sweet Potato | 1 sweet potato, salt, | Bake until tender. | 100 calories, 0g fat | 1 potato | 45 minutes |

| | cinnamon | | | | |
|---|---|---|---|---|---|
| 15. Pumpkin Smoothie | ½ cup canned pumpkin, 1 cup almond milk, honey | Blend ingredients until smooth. | 200 calories, 3g fat | 1 cup | 5 minutes |

This table provides a variety of snacks, from smoothies and desserts to more savory options, tailored to be gentle on the stomach for those with gastroparesis. Each recipe focuses on minimizing fiber and fat while providing sufficient nutrition and energy.

# Recipes for GastroparesisFriendly Meals

Here's a table featuring 15 gastroparesis-friendly recipes that focus on easy-to-digest ingredients and minimal fiber content, which are essential considerations for anyone managing this condition. These recipes are designed to be nutritious while keeping symptoms in check.

| Recipe Name | Ingredients | Instructions | Nutritional Information (per serving) | Serving Size | Cooking Time |
|---|---|---|---|---|---|
| 1. Chicken & Rice Soup | - 1 cup cooked white rice<br>- 1 cup cooked, shredded chicken | - Combine all ingredients in a large pot.<br>- Heat to a boil and | Calories: 200<br>Fat: 3g<br>Protein: 15g | 1 cup | 25 mins |

| | <br>- 4 cups chicken broth | then simmer for 20 minutes. | | | |
|---|---|---|---|---|---|
| 2. Mashed Potatoes | - 4 large potatoes, peeled<br>- 1/4 cup milk<br>- 2 tbsp butter | - Boil potatoes until tender.<br>- Mash with milk and butter until smooth. | Calories: 150<br>Fat: 4g<br>Carbs: 26g | 1/2 cup | 30 mins |
| 3. Banana Smoothie | - 1 banana<br>- 1 cup low-fat milk<br>- 1 | - Blend all ingredients until smooth. | Calories: 180<br>Fat: 1g<br>Protein: 5g | 1 glass | 5 mins |

| | tbsp honey | | | | |
| --- | --- | --- | --- | --- | --- |
| 4. Poache d Fish | - 1 fillet white fish<br>- 1 lemon<br>- 1 tsp olive oil | - Place fish in a skillet with a thin layer of water and lemon juice.<br>- Cover and simmer until fish flakes easily. | Calories: 120<br>Fat: 2g<br>Protein: 20g | 1 fillet | 15 mins |
| 5. Apple Sauce | - 4 apples, peeled and cored< | - Combi ne ingredie nts in a | Calories: 100<br>Fat: 0g<br> | 1/2 cup | 25 mins |

| | br>-<br>1/2 cup<br>water<<br>br>- 1<br>tsp<br>cinnam<br>on | pot.<br>>-<br>Cook<br>until<br>apples<br>are soft,<br>then<br>mash. | Carbs:<br>25g | | |
| --- | --- | --- | --- | --- | --- |
| 6.<br>Oatmea<br>l<br>Porridg<br>e | - 1 cup<br>rolled<br>oats<br>>- 2<br>cups<br>water<<br>br>- 1<br>tsp<br>sugar | - Bring<br>water to<br>a<br>boil.<br>>- Add<br>oats<br>and<br>simmer<br>until<br>cooked.<br>Stir in<br>sugar. | Calories<br>:<br>150<br>>Fat:<br>3g<br>Carbs:<br>27g | 1 bowl | 10 mins |
| 7. Egg<br>Custard | - 2<br>eggs<br>>- 1<br>cup<br>milk<b | - Whisk<br>eggs,<br>milk,<br>and<br>sugar.< | Calories<br>:<br>130<br>>Fat:<br>5g<br> | 1<br>serving | 45 mins |

| | | | | | |
|---|---|---|---|---|---|
| | r>- 2 tbsp sugar | br>- Bake in a water bath at 325°F until set. | Protein: 6g | | |
| 8. Vegetable Broth | - 1 carrot, peeled<br>- 1 celery stalk<br>- 4 cups water | - Simmer all ingredients until flavors meld.<br>- Strain out solids. | Calories: 40<br>Fat: 0g<br>Carbs: 9g | 1 cup | 30 mins |
| 9. Avocado Puree | - 1 ripe avocado<br>- 1/2 tsp lime juice<b | - Blend avocado with lime juice and salt | Calories: 240<br>Fat: 22g<br | 1/2 cup | 5 mins |

| | r>- Salt to taste | until smooth . | >Carbs: 13g | | |
|---|---|---|---|---|---|
| 10. Baked Custard | - 3 eggs<br>- 2 cups milk<br>- 1/4 cup sugar | - Mix ingredients and pour into ramekins.<br> - Bake at 300°F in a water bath until set. | Calories: 180<br>Fat: 6g<br>Protein: 9g | 1 ramekin | 50 mins |
| 11. Cream of Wheat | - 1/2 cup cream of wheat<br>- 2 cups | - Heat milk to a boil.<br>- Slowly stir in | Calories: 160<br>Fat: 2g<br>Carbs: 32g | 1 bowl | 15 mins |

|  | milk<br>- 2 tbsp sugar | cream of wheat and sugar.<br>- Simmer until thickened. |  |  |  |
| 12. Rice Pudding | - 1/2 cup cooked white rice<br>- 1 cup milk<br>- 1/4 cup sugar | - Mix rice, milk, and sugar in a pot.<br>- Cook over low heat until thick. | Calories: 150<br>Fat: 2g<br>Carbs: 28g | 1/2 cup | 25 mins |

| 13. Ginger Tea | - 1 inch ginger root, peeled<br>- 1 cup water | - Simmer ginger in water for 10 minutes.<br>- Strain and serve hot. | Calories: 10<br>Fat: 0g<br>Carbs: 2g | 1 cup | 15 mins |
| 14. Flan | - 3 eggs<br>- 1 can condensed milk<br>- 1 can evaporated milk<br>- 1/2 cup sugar | - Mix all ingredients and pour into a mold.<br>- Bake in a water bath at 350°F until set. | Calories: 280<br>Fat: 8g<br>Protein: 7g | 1 slice | 60 mins |

| 15. Chicken Puree | - 1 cup cooked, shredded chicken<br>- 1/2 cup chicken broth<br>- Salt and pepper to taste | - Blend chicken with broth until smooth.<br>- Season with salt and pepper and warm before serving. | Calories: 140<br>Fat: 3g<br>Protein: 20g | 1/2 cup | 10 mins |
| --- | --- | --- | --- | --- | --- |

These recipes aim to provide balanced nutrition while minimizing the risk of aggravating gastroparesis symptoms. They incorporate easily digestible foods with low fiber content to ensure that meals are as stomach-friendly as possible.

# Chapter 4: Foods to Avoid

## Foods That Aggravate Gastroparesis

Below is a table that details foods known to aggravate gastroparesis symptoms, explaining why they should be avoided. This guide helps individuals with gastroparesis make informed decisions about their diet to minimize discomfort and manage symptoms more effectively.

| Food Group | Examples | Reason to Avoid |
| --- | --- | --- |
| **High-Fiber Vegetables** | - Broccoli<br>- Cabbage<br>- Cauliflower | These vegetables contain high levels of insoluble fiber, which is difficult for the stomach to break down, potentially leading to blockages or severe slowdowns in gastric emptying. |
| **Legumes** | - Beans<br>- Lentils<br>- Peas | Legumes are high in fiber and can |

| | | ferment in the stomach, causing excessive bloating and discomfort, further slowing down gastric emptying. |
| **Whole Grains** | - Whole wheat bread<br>- Brown rice<br>- Quinoa | Whole grains are rich in fiber which can be challenging to digest and can remain in the stomach for a long time, exacerbating symptoms of gastroparesis. |
| **Tough Meats** | - Steak<br>- Pork chops<br>- Sausages | Tough, fatty meats require more gastric effort to digest and can significantly delay the emptying process, leading to increased symptoms. |

| Fried Foods | - French fries<br>- Fried chicken<br>- Donuts | Fried foods are high in fat which slows down stomach emptying. They can also be greasy, adding to the difficulty of digestion and increasing the risk of gastroesophageal reflux. |
| Dairy Products | - Cream<br>- Ice cream<br>- Full-fat cheese | High-fat dairy products can slow gastric emptying. They may also contribute to the formation of bezoars, which are solid masses of food that form in the stomach and can block digestion. |

| Raw Fruits | - Apples<br>- Berries<br>- Oranges | Raw fruits are typically high in fiber, particularly in their skins, which are tough to digest. They can also contribute to blockage and slow gastric processing. |
| **Sugary Foods** | - Candy<br>- Cakes<br>- Cookies | Sugary foods can cause rapid fluctuations in blood sugar levels, which can affect digestion negatively. They often lack nutritional value and can replace more digestible and nutritious foods. |
| **Carbonated Beverages** | - Soda<br>- Sparkling water | These can introduce excess air into the |

| | | stomach, increase bloating, and exacerbate symptoms of nausea and feeling overly full. |
| --- | --- | --- |
| **Spicy Foods** | - Hot peppers<br>- Salsa<br>- Spicy curries | Spicy foods can irritate the stomach lining, exacerbate symptoms of gastroparesis, and lead to discomfort such as heartburn and gastric distress. |
| **Alcohol** | - Beer<br>- Wine<br>- Spirits | Alcohol can irritate the stomach lining and increase symptoms of gastroparesis. It also dehydrates the body and can interfere with medications used |

| | | |
|---|---|---|
| | | to treat gastroparesis. |
| **Caffeinated Beverages** | - Coffee<br>- Black tea<br>- Energy drinks | Caffeine can stimulate acid production in the stomach, leading to increased discomfort and potentially worsening gastroparesis symptoms. It can also disrupt sleep patterns. |

This table highlights the types of foods that can exacerbate the symptoms of gastroparesis by increasing the burden on the stomach's already compromised ability to digest and empty its contents effectively. People with gastroparesis are generally advised to avoid these foods to manage their symptoms better and improve their quality of life.

# Common Triggers and How to Identify Them

Below is a table detailing common triggers for gastroparesis symptoms, including specific foods to avoid and explanations of why these items can exacerbate the condition. Identifying and understanding these triggers is crucial for managing gastroparesis effectively.

| Common Trigger | Why to Avoid | How to Identify |
| --- | --- | --- |
| **High Fiber Vegetables** | Fiber can be difficult to digest and may slow gastric emptying. It can also form bezoars. | Avoid vegetables like broccoli, cauliflower, corn, and legumes. Look for terms like "high fiber" on labels or choose vegetables that are more easily digestible, such as well-cooked carrots. |
| **Fatty Foods** | Fat slows down the digestive process, which can worsen | Limit intake of fried foods, full-fat dairy products, |

| | gastroparesis symptoms. | and fatty cuts of meat. Opt for low-fat or fat-free options when available. |
| --- | --- | --- |
| **Raw Fruits and Vegetables** | Raw produce is harder to digest, potentially leading to increased symptoms. | Cook fruits and vegetables to aid digestibility. Avoid salads and whole, raw fruit. Peel skins and remove seeds as they are harder to digest. |
| **Carbonated Beverages** | These can cause bloating and increase gastric pressure, aggravating symptoms. | Choose non-carbonated, caffeine-free, and low-sugar drinks. Always read beverage labels to avoid carbonated options. |
| **Alcohol** | Alcohol can irritate the stomach lining and | Avoid alcoholic beverages entirely, especially those |

| | affect gastric motility. | high in sugar or mixed with carbonated mixers. |
| **Spicy Foods** | Spices can irritate the stomach and exacerbate nausea and vomiting. | Avoid foods with hot spices, pepper, or chili. Opt for bland, non-spiced foods. Always check ingredient lists for hidden spices. |
| **Caffeine** | Caffeine can stimulate acid production and lead to stomach discomfort. | Limit or avoid coffee, tea, and some soft drinks. Look for caffeine-free alternatives and read labels to ensure beverages do not contain caffeine. |
| **Chocolate** | Contains caffeine and fats, which can slow digestion and | Avoid chocolate and chocolate-based |

| | | |
|---|---|---|
| | increase symptoms. | desserts as they typically combine high fat and caffeine. Choose non-chocolate sweets if desired, checking for low fat content. |
| **Nuts and Seeds** | These are high in fat and fiber, both of which can complicate digestion in gastroparesis. | Avoid all types of nuts and seeds, and foods containing them, such as certain breads or desserts. Look for smooth, nut-free spreads as alternatives. |
| **Whole Grains** | High in fiber, whole grains can be difficult to digest and slow gastric emptying. | Choose refined grains like white bread, pasta, and rice instead of whole grain options. Carefully read labels to avoid |

| | | whole grain products. |
| --- | --- | --- |

For those managing gastroparesis, understanding and avoiding these common triggers can significantly reduce symptoms and improve digestive function. It's important to note that everyone's response to different foods can vary, so maintaining a food diary to track symptoms in relation to specific foods consumed can be a helpful tool in managing this condition effectively.

# Tips for Eliminating Problematic Foods

Here's a table offering insights on identifying and eliminating problematic foods from the diet of individuals with gastroparesis. It lists specific types of foods to avoid due to their potential to exacerbate symptoms, along with strategies for effectively removing these foods from daily consumption and the reasons for doing so.

| Problematic Food Group | Tips for Elimination | Reasons to Avoid |
| --- | --- | --- |
| **Raw Vegetables** | Start by reducing intake gradually and monitor symptoms. Replace with cooked vegetables that are easier to digest. | Raw vegetables are high in insoluble fiber, which can be difficult to digest, leading to increased symptoms like bloating and nausea. |
| **Fibrous Fruits** | Peel fruits to reduce fiber content and choose canned or | Similar to vegetables, fibrous fruits can slow down gastric emptying and |

| | | |
|---|---|---|
| | cooked fruits instead of raw. | exacerbate symptoms. |
| **Whole Grains** | Replace whole grains with refined grains like white bread and plain pasta, which are easier on the stomach. | Whole grains contain a high amount of fiber that can delay stomach emptying and complicate digestion. |
| **Fatty Meats** | Opt for lean cuts of meat and use cooking methods like boiling or steaming instead of frying. | Fats can greatly slow down the digestive process, causing discomfort and increasing symptoms of gastroparesis. |
| **Legumes** | Eliminate legumes gradually and opt for low-fiber protein sources like eggs or tofu. | Legumes are typically high in fiber and can be difficult to digest, leading to increased gastrointestinal distress. |

| | | |
|---|---|---|
| **Dairy Products** | Introduce lactose-free or low-fat dairy options if dairy is problematic; monitor symptoms to gauge tolerance. | High-fat dairy products can slow down stomach emptying. Lactose may also cause symptoms if there's an intolerance. |
| **Fried Foods** | Avoid all forms of fried foods and replace them with baked or steamed alternatives. | Fried foods are high in fat, which can inhibit gastric emptying and lead to increased symptoms. |
| **Spicy Foods** | Gradually reduce the spice level in foods to determine tolerance levels and opt for mild flavors. | Spicy foods can irritate the stomach lining, potentially worsening gastroparesis symptoms. |
| **Carbonated Beverages** | Replace carbonated drinks with flat, | Carbonation can cause bloating and gas, leading to |

| | | |
|---|---|---|
| | non-carbonated options like herbal teas or water. | discomfort and increased pressure on the stomach. |
| **Alcoholic Beverages** | Eliminate alcohol from the diet entirely as it can interfere with digestion and the medications often used for treatment. | Alcohol can irritate the stomach lining and affect the rate at which the stomach empties. |
| **Nuts and Seeds** | Avoid nuts and seeds as they are high in fats and difficult to digest; opt for smooth nut butters if needed. | Their high fiber and fat content make them particularly challenging for a stomach affected by gastroparesis to process efficiently. |
| **Sweets and Sugars** | Limit high-sugar foods as they can lead to spikes in blood sugar levels, complicating | Sugary foods can cause rapid gastric emptying, which may not be ideal for gastroparesis management, |

| | gastroparesis management. | especially in diabetics. |
| --- | --- | --- |

By carefully eliminating or substituting these foods with easier-to-digest options, individuals with gastroparesis can manage their symptoms more effectively and improve their overall digestive health. Each change in the diet should be monitored to see how it affects symptoms, allowing for more personalized dietary management of gastroparesis.

# Conclusion

Managing gastroparesis through diet is a critical aspect of improving quality of life for those affected by this condition. By carefully selecting foods that are easier to digest and preparing them in ways that facilitate smoother gastric processing, individuals can significantly reduce the severity of their symptoms. It is important to remember that while the diet does not cure gastroparesis, it helps to manage and mitigate the symptoms associated with delayed gastric emptying.

Adhering to a gastroparesis-friendly diet often requires eliminating or significantly reducing the intake of foods that are high in fats, fibers, and certain complex carbohydrates. This doesn't just help in reducing the symptoms like nausea, vomiting, and bloating, but it also aids in preventing the formation of bezoars, which are hardened masses of undigested food that can block the gastrointestinal system. Opting for cooked over raw vegetables, choosing low-fat protein sources, and consuming refined grains can all contribute to a more manageable digestive process.

The importance of meal frequency and size cannot be overstated for those with gastroparesis. Eating smaller, more frequent meals helps prevent the stomach from becoming overly full, which can exacerbate gastroparesis symptoms. This approach not only helps in managing the volume of food that needs to be digested but also stabilizes blood sugar levels, which is particularly beneficial for patients who also suffer from diabetes.

Hydration is another crucial element in managing gastroparesis, as adequate fluid intake helps to facilitate digestion and prevent dehydration, especially in those who experience frequent vomiting. However, liquids should be consumed separately from solids to avoid overfilling the stomach during meals. Opting for non-carbonated and non-alcoholic beverages is advisable to minimize any potential for gastric irritation.

Consultation with healthcare professionals, including gastroenterologists and dietitians, is essential when managing gastroparesis through diet. These experts can provide tailored advice based on individual health needs and help monitor the progression of the condition. A dietitian, in particular, can assist in creating meal plans that meet nutritional needs while considering the limitations imposed by gastroparesis, ensuring that patients receive balanced nutrition despite their dietary restrictions.

As research continues and more is understood about gastroparesis, dietary recommendations may evolve. Therefore, staying informed about the latest findings and treatment strategies is vital for those managing this condition. This can involve participating in patient support groups, staying in regular contact with healthcare providers, and keeping abreast of new research through credible sources.

Ultimately, the goal of any dietary strategy for gastroparesis is to improve the patient's ability to process food efficiently and comfortably. While adjustments to diet and lifestyle can be challenging, the benefits in terms of symptom relief and improved digestive function are substantial. Careful management and adherence to a well-constructed gastroparesis diet can lead to a significant enhancement in life quality, allowing individuals to manage their condition more effectively and enjoy a broader range of activities with fewer gastrointestinal disturbances.